SECRETS
OF STRESS
MANAGEMENT

do it yourself now without even a coach

by Ayoub Sbai

Book Cover by Ayoub Sbai
edition 2023

TABLE OF
CONTENTS

INTRODUCTION

"**I**'m SO stressed out," you seem to hear almost daily from everyone you know. There are many pressures in the world nowadays. These pressures lead to stress and anxiety, and we are frequently ill-prepared to handle the stressors that result in anxiety and other unpleasant emotions that may lead to illness. ill, literally.

The numbers are astounding. An anxiety condition affects one in eight Americans between the ages of 18 and 54. Over 19 million people in all! Anxiety disorders are the second most common mental health issue among American women, after alcohol and drug abuse, according to research from the National Institute of Mental Health.

Compared to men, women experience worry and stress almost twice as frequently. In terms of prevalence, anxiety disorders outnumber depression as the most prevalent mental illness in America. The most prevalent mental health condition affecting persons over 65 is anxiety. Each year, anxiety problems cost the United States $46.6 billion. Patients with anxiety typically see five doctors before receiving a correct diagnosis.

Unfortunately, anxiety and stress often coexist. In actuality, anxiety is one of the main signs of stress. Additionally, stress is directly or indirectly responsible for 80 percent of all illnesses.

Stress is actually more harmful than we previously realized. Although you've surely heard that stress can raise blood pressure, raising the risk of a stroke in the distant future, a recent health insurance pamphlet indicated that stress-related problems accounted for 90% of visits to a primary care physician.

According to Health Psychology magazine, ongoing stress might hinder the immune system's ability to operate normally. Additionally, studies have shown that people who are under stress are more prone to getting sick and are also more likely to develop allergic, autoimmune, or cardiovascular diseases.

According to medical professionals, the digestive and immune systems, as well as other bodily processes not necessary for survival, shut down under prolonged stress. People get sick because of this, he claims. Psychosomatic illness, a disease with an emotional or psychological component, is also very common.

Additionally, stress frequently causes people to react in unhealthy ways, like smoking, drinking alcohol, eating poorly, or engaging in inactive lifestyles. In addition to the wear and tear caused by the stress itself, this harms the body.

Stress is a natural part of life. Maintaining our health and wellbeing depends entirely on how we respond to it. Life is full of pressures, and those pressures lead to stress. You must accept that stress will always be a part of your life, but you can learn coping mechanisms to transform it into a more positive experience.

I remember thinking when I first received the task of writing this book, "Sure, you can get rid of stress and anxiety by locking yourself in a room and never talking to anyone again." But a book like that wouldn't be very educational, would it?

Stress-related anxiety disorders have plagued me for a long time. Despite constantly learning new topics and coping techniques, I feel like I have learnt how to deal with that in some ways. In order to give you tools that will aid you in difficult situations, I've blended some of my own experiences with guidance from professionals in this book.

I've also provided several strategies for dealing with the crippling anxiety and panic episodes that many individuals experience. I've discovered some incredible stuff while doing research for this book, and I can't wait to share it with you. Let's look at how to get rid of tension and worry from your life because I've learned so much myself!

WHY ARE WE FELLING SO STRESSED OUT?

We are in extremely stressful and challenging times, and nothing appears to be getting any better. Even though life can often feel incredibly difficult and unfair, we manage to push through, day after day, hoping and praying that things will get better soon.

But the world is getting weirder, more unpredictable, and more stressful on a daily basis. These days, nothing feels secure. There are record numbers of people who are in debt. Many people are losing their jobs, homes, health, and occasionally even their sanity. There are far too many people who seem to live with worry, sadness, and anxiety.

The Age of Anxiety appears to have arrived. In fact, Time magazine loudly and clearly announced this as the featured subject in that issue on one of its covers in 2002. Many of us appear to lead lives marked by perpetual anxiety and concern as a result of the strain and uncertainty that come with living in the twenty-first century.

This ongoing anxiety and stress seemed to get worse after the September 11 terrorist strikes. In fact, many individuals say they are still terrified that something of that size could occur again, possibly closer to them, four years later.

We are constantly exposed to upsetting visuals and tales when we turn on the news or open a newspaper. We start to doubt where we are safe. Never before have we had such easy access to so much information as we do in this era of information.

The economy is another source of stress. Both our nation and many Americans are in debt. Many Americans now work in monotonous and unsatisfactory occupations as a result of rising gas prices, exorbitant housing costs, and even the cost of food. They work these tasks in order to support themselves. Nowadays, having a stable job is more crucial than having a dream one.

The stress is increased when there are more women in the workforce. So many women believe they must be the breadwinner, the housekeeper, the mother, the wife, the daughter, and the sister. The only issue with that is that some women simply don't carve out time for themselves, which contributes to their chronic stress.

Even young children can experience stress and anxiety. Teenagers who want to attend colleges often push themselves academically to try and get scholarships so they can attend institutions with rising tuition costs.

In addition to all of that, they find themselves having to work part-time jobs to pay for extras that their parents can no longer afford. Peer pressure makes the situation into a true pressure cooker!

With the help of cell phones, the internet, palm pilots, blackberries, and ipods, we are constantly on the move and reachable. We no longer set aside time to unwind and relish life. why not Of course we should!

We feel under pressure to carry out these actions because we believe we MUST rather than because we WANT to. People find it difficult to just say "No" far too frequently. By not speaking just one simple word, we accumulate unnecessary duties and expectations, which causes us anxiety.

Every one of us will come across circumstances that could lead to worry or anxiety. The causes are too numerous to list, but some of them include purchasing a home, having overnight guests (in-laws!), being bullied, attending exams, caring for children, handling finances, having marital problems, traveling, etc.

It's "natural" to experience stress in daily life. It doesn't actually become a problem until it seems to rule our life.

Everyone will feel pressured for different reasons depending on the circumstances. Generally speaking, we become anxious or tense when we don't feel in control of a situation and we can feel its grip tightening around us.

The solution is to try to change this and regain control if stress is brought on by our lack of feeling in control of a situation. You can, which is wonderful news!

You already possess all of the resources required to beat stress and the resulting worry. The issue is that because we sometimes feel so out of control, we frequently fail to recognize that we are in charge. But you only need to use the available tools.

Let's first examine the obstacles we erect that prohibit us from achieving health and overcoming our anxiety and tension.

BLOCKING BEHAVIOURS THAT MAINTAIN STRESS

There is no doubt that you engage in three compulsive behaviors that have hampered your recovery and keep you from leading a stress-free life. Recognizing these challenges can be the first step in overcoming the problems brought on by excessive stress. Obsession with negativity is the first. Being compulsively negative is defined as having a tendency to be "negative" about people, places, situations, and other facets of your life.

It's possible to think of phrases like "I can't do this!" or "No one understands!" or "Nothing ever works!" Even though you may not be aware of it, your "sour grapes" attitude prevents you from understanding what it's like to view life from a positive perspective and appreciate the beauty in yourself and those around you. There is a vast universe full of fun and inspiring ideas for you. Compulsive perfectionism is the next. Obsessive perfectionism involves trying to do everything "just so," even if doing so results in anxiety for you. You might catch yourself telling yourself things like, "I have to finish this perfectly or I'll fail!" or "If I'm not precise, people will be mad at me." Again, even though you may be completely unaware of this behavior, it has a negative impact on your ability to enjoy activities without getting "uptight" or "stressed." The final category of analysis is OCD. When you are obsessed with analysis, you find that you want to come back to a task or an issue time and time again. One would think of statements like, "I need to read something over, study it, and know it inside and out...or else I can't relax!" or "Things go wrong if I relax and stop double-checking them!"

Although the capacity for analytical thought is a wonderful trait, if it takes over your life, you won't have time to stop and appreciate the beauty of the world around you because you'll be too busy trying to make sense of everything and everyone. Understanding this kind of behavior is one of the most important steps to letting go of tension and taking full control of your anxiety.

If you notice yourself engaging in any of the aforementioned "Blocking Behaviors," you have two options to help yourself. Start by inquiring about your negative, whiny, or difficult personality traits from the people you know, love, and trust.

You might have trouble hearing what I'm saying because the truth is frequently very painful.

However, you will gain a priceless perspective on how people see you and be fully aware of those perceptions. Accept their advice as helpful information, and have faith in your ability to gain a lot of knowledge from what they have to say.

Keep a journal to track your "blocking behaviors" and spot trends in your behavior. Even if you dislike writing, you can make quick notes every day in a notebook or journal. The best part is that you'll begin to spot behavioral patterns that reveal how you're delaying treating your anxiety. But you must first identify these blocks in order to proceed to the "healing" step and get rid of your stress and anxiety. Later in the book, we'll give you some fantastic stress-relieving strategies. Many people think that the phrases stress and anxiety are equivalent. You see, the reverse is true! ANXIETY OR STRESS

Contrary to popular assumption, stress and anxiety are not synonymous. The pressures we experience in life lead to stress, which is caused by the hormone adrenaline being released. An extended period of the hormone's presence can lead to depression, an increase in blood pressure, and other undesirable changes and outcomes.

Anxiety is one among these adverse consequences. When a person has anxiety, fear takes the place of all other emotions, including concern and apprehension, leaving them isolated and jittery. Chest aches, lightheadedness, shortness of breath, and panic episodes are further symptoms.

An existing stressor or stressors are what cause

stress. Stress that persists after the stressor has passed is anxiety. Any circumstance or thinking that makes you feel irritated, furious, worried, or even anxious might cause stress. Not everything that stresses out one person will necessarily stress out another.

Anxiety is a state of trepidation or worry that nearly often comes with a sense of impending disaster. The fact that you may not always be aware of the cause of your discomfort can make you feel worse.

Stress is the way that our bodies and thoughts respond to something that breaks the equilibrium of our daily lives; an example of stress is the reaction that we experience when we feel threatened or scared. The hormone adrenaline, which activates our body's defense mechanisms and causes our hearts to race, blood pressure to increase, muscles to tense, and eye pupils to widen, is released by our adrenal glands during stressful situations.

Your pulse rate increasing is one of the main signs of increased stress, but having a normal pulse doesn't mean you're not anxious. You may notice symptoms of stress such as persistent aches and pains, palpitations, worry, chronic exhaustion, sobbing, overeating or undereating, recurrent infections, and a decline in your sexual desire.

Naturally, we do not always respond in such severe ways to stress, and we are not always under as much pressure or dread when we are faced with a difficult circumstance.

Stress affects some people more than others; for some, even routine daily decisions seem impossible. For them, choosing what to eat for supper or what to buy at the supermarket presents a seemingly insurmountable challenge. On the other hand, some people appear to flourish under strain by becoming extremely productive while being propelled by the pressure.

According to research, women who have children have greater blood levels of stress-related hormones than women who do not. Does this imply that women without children don't go through stressful times? Without a doubt!

It implies that women who are childless may not suffer stress as frequently or to the same degree as women who are parents. This means that scheduling time for yourself is especially crucial for women who are raising children because once your stress level is lower, you will be better able to support your kids and handle the daily challenges of being a parent.

On the other side, anxiety is a sense of unease. Everybody feels it when they are in a stressful circumstance, as right before an exam or an interview, or when they are experiencing a health concern. When facing something challenging or risky, it's acceptable to feel apprehensive, and mild anxiety might even be a good thing.

But for many people, anxiety makes daily life difficult. Excessive anxiety frequently coexists with psychiatric disorders like depression. When anxiety is exceedingly intense or persistent, occurs in the absence of a stressful incident, or interferes with regular tasks like going to work, it is deemed abnormal.

The brain sends signals to various body parts in order to get them ready for the "fight or flight" reaction, which results in the physical symptoms of anxiety. The body's organs that function faster include the heart, lungs, and others Adrenaline and other stress hormones are also released by the brain. The following are typical signs of excessive anxiety:

•Fear of going "crazy"
•Dry mouth;
•rapid heartbeat or palpitations;
•insomnia;
•irritability or rage;
•inability to focus;
•feeling unreal and out of control of your actions (also known as depersonalization);

There are numerous techniques to induce anxiety. It goes without saying that stress in your life can cause you to have uneasy thoughts. Many persons with anxiety problems spend a lot of time worrying excessively. This can be worry over anything, including your health, your career, or global issues.

Certain substances, both illegal and legal, can cause withdrawal symptoms or side effects that can resemble anxiety symptoms.

Caffeine, alcohol, nicotine, cold treatments, decongestants, bronchodilators for asthma, tricyclic antidepressants, cocaine, amphetamines, diet pills, ADHD meds, and thyroid medications are some examples of these substances.

Stress or anxiety can also be brought on by an unhealthy diet, such as one with insufficient vitamin B12 levels. Performance anxiety is linked to certain circumstances, such as taking a test or giving a public presentation. A stressful incident like war, physical or sexual abuse, or a natural disaster can cause post-traumatic stress disorder (PTSD), a stress disorder.

An adrenal gland tumor known as a pheochromocytoma may occasionally be the root of anxiety. The hormones that trigger anxiety-related thoughts, feelings, and behaviors are overproduced as a result of this.

Although nervousness can be a little frightening, what's much scarier is how much stress and worry can contribute to depression. I am well aware that dealing with depression can be a lifelong struggle, but the good news is that everything can be controlled!

So let's take a few quick tests to determine whether you have an excessive amount of stress, anxiety, or sadness.

QUIZ TIME!

Please be aware that we are not medical specialists before you continue. This material has been verified but is in no way intended to be a comprehensive diagnostic tool. These tests are merely guides to assist you in identifying any issues you may have and being able to successfully address those issues.

Let's start with determining whether you might be depressed because it can be the most serious of our themes. Remember that everyone experiences "blue" days occasionally. The fact that the symptoms develop gradually distinguishes clinical depression from mere melancholy. They are persistent and have the potential to negatively impact your life; they don't come and go. Consider the following queries. If you have had these feelings consistently during the past two weeks, select yes.

1. Do you feel down all the time?
2. Do you lack the motivation to carry out routine tasks like take a shower, clean the house, or prepare dinner?
3. Do people frequently comment on your irritability?

4. Do you find it difficult to focus?

5. Do your loved ones and friends make you feel lonely, even when they are present?

6. Have you stopped enjoying your favorite pastimes?

7. Do you ever feel useless, hopeless, or guilty without any justification?

8. Do you struggle to fall asleep and are perpetually tired?

9. Has your weight considerably changed?

If "Yes" is your response to five or more of these inquiries, you may be experiencing clinical depression. You should look for medical assistance from a professional, such as a doctor or therapist. There are numerous drugs available that can treat depression.

When I started taking an anti-depressant, I tried to hide my own depression but I couldn't believe what a difference just one pill a day made! If you believe you are depressed, take action right away. It helped me escape the "black hole" I had become trapped in and helped me enjoy life again. You should be content. Let's check to see if you're overly stressed out, though, since this book is about stress and anxiety. Consider the following:

1. Do you frequently worry and engage in critical self-talk?

2. Do you find it difficult to focus?

3. Are you irritable and quick to react?

4. Do you frequently get neck or head pain?

5. Are you a teeth-grinder?

6. Do you experience anxiety, depression, or regular overwhelm?

Do you overeat, drink excessively, smoke, argue, or use other harmful coping mechanisms to escape yourself and life?

8. Do you find that simple pleasures don't satisfy you?

9. Do you occasionally lose your temper at little issues?

You have excessive stress in your life if you can "Yes" to the majority of these questions. The good news is that by purchasing this book, you will gain access to a wealth of useful stress-reduction strategies. However, we'll discuss that later. Now let's talk about anxiety.

1. Do you ever shake, have a racing heart, or have shortness of breath when you're at rest?

2. Do you worry about losing your mind or going crazy?

3. Do you shy away from social situations out of fear?

4. Do you have any object phobias?

5. Do you worry that you'll be stuck somewhere or in an uncomfortable circumstance?

6. Do you worry about leaving your house?

7. Do you get recurring ideas or visions that won't go away?

8. Do you find yourself doing the same things over and over again?

9. Do you frequently replay a distressing prior event?

More than four "Yes" responses to these questions may suggest an anxiety problem.

Your general health may be jeopardized if you experience depression, high levels of stress, or excessive worry, thus it is imperative that you take action right away to overcome these issues.

Numerous physical and psychological aspects of our bodies are impacted by stress and anxiety. Because stress and anxiety cause changes in our bodies' chemical makeup, they are linked to cancer and other deadly diseases.

Stress and anxiety don't have to control your life; all it takes is discipline and a structured schedule. It will be very helpful to avoid consuming anything that you cannot handle. Recognize your restrictions and abide by them. Never overwork yourself. Simply attempt to cross the border a single inch at a time.

Without putting your health at risk, you can live a successful, fulfilling life and career. If not, you are not only killing yourself but also your loved ones, friends, and everyone else in your vicinity.

Life is certain to be stressful at times. It can be both physical and mental, and a lot of the time, pressures from daily life can cause it. There are differences between how each person manages stress.

However, if stress is not managed, it can lead to

behavioral, mental, and physical issues that can harm your relationships at work and in your personal life as well as your health.

As previously stated, panic attacks can result from stress and anxiety. Having a panic attack can be a serious issue, as I can attest from personal experience. Let's delve a little more into that topic.

PANIC ATTACKS

The unfortunate result of experiencing excessive stress and anxiety is that your body will respond to the situation physically. It appears as though your body is urging you to take a short break. It's anything but restful when you're experiencing a panic attack, though. While my husband and I were returning from a St. Louis Rams football game, I experienced my first panic attack. I started to feel a little "off" when we were about 30 miles from our house. My heart seemed to be beating at a speed of 90 miles per hour, I was having problems breathing, and I felt separated from my body. I parked the van by the side of the road and got out in the hope that I might "walk it off." It didn't, though. No matter what I did, I was unable to get a breath. I thought I was going to die. I can still hear myself pleading, "Please not now. I'm not prepared. It was gruesome. The good news is that I obviously wasn't going to die! But that evening marked the start of a terrible exploration of how my body responded to high levels of stress and anxiety. Since then, I've experienced a lot of panic attacks, but I've also developed the ability to spot and manage them when they do. It's a lot better than it was, even though I can't always fully control it and occasionally experience full-blown panic. Let's now examine the warning signs of a potential panic attack. The list that follows identifies warning signs of impending panic attacks.

Palpitations,
a racing heart, an elevated heart rate,
sweating,
trembling,
shaking, shortness of breath,
a feeling of choking,
chest pain or discomfort,
nausea, or stomach cramps,
de-realization (a sense of disassociation from reality),
fear of losing control or going crazy,
fear of passing away,
numbness or tingling in your face and limbs,
chills,
or hot flashes are all symptoms of menopause.

You'd be surprised at how many patients arrive at the emergency room of the hospital absolutely certain that they are having a heart attack only to learn that it is actually a panic attack. They are that serious!
When you have a panic attack, it can be very difficult for your loved ones to comprehend or even picture what you are going through. They might become impatient with you, tell you to "get over it," or

suspect you of being a fake. If you show them the following scenario, it might be helpful.

At the grocery store, there is a line. Even though you've been waiting for a while, there is only one more customer before you reach the cashier. What the heck was that?

Your chest tightens, an unpleasant sensation develops in your throat, you start to feel suddenly short of breath, and, what do you know, your heart begins to skip a beat. "God, please don't be here."

You quickly survey the area to see if it poses a threat. There are four hostile faces behind you and one in front of you. You feel as though pins and needles are stabbing you through your left arm, you start to feel a little lightheaded, and then fear explodes as you prepare for the worst. A panic attack is about to happen to you.

You are now certain that this will be a significant event. Now you need to pay attention. You are aware of how to handle this, or at least you think you are! Start inhaling deeply while exhaling through your mouth.

Breathe in, repeat the word "Relax," while thinking soothing ideas, and then exhale. However, it doesn't seem to be helping; in fact, focusing just on breathing makes you feel self-conscious and more tense.

Perhaps if you simply attempt to relax your muscles. Hold the tension in both shoulders for 10 seconds, then let go. Try it one more. Nope, there hasn't changed. The anxiety is getting worse, and the lack of effective coping mechanisms makes your terror much worse. If only your family or a close friend were there to support you, you could feel more at ease handling this circumstance.

Your body is now buzzing with unpleasant sensations, the adrenaline in your system is really rushing, and you are experiencing the dreadful feeling of losing all control of your emotions. Nobody nearby has any clue of the extreme terror you are going through. They view it as just another ordinary day and another interminably long grocery line.

You understand you have no other choices. Time to leave now. As it is now your moment to pay, you remove yourself from the line while still looking ashamed. As you leave your purchases behind and make your way to the door, the cashier is staring at you perplexed.

You need some alone time; there is no time for justifications. You exit the store and get in your car to drive home by yourself. You ponder whether this was the major incident. The person you fear will make you physically and mentally exhausted. The panic eases ten minutes later. How on earth are you going to get through the rest of your day when it's only 11:00 in the morning?

The above scenario probably sounds very familiar if you frequently experience panic or anxiety attacks. Even simply reading it might have caused anxiety and fear. In fact, even writing it was challenging for me.

You could experience panic and anxiety in different situations. The physical sensations might be a little different. It's crucial to understand that panic attacks are really real to the people experiencing them, and they shouldn't ever be ignored.

One evening at home, I was alone and I was watching one of my favorite shows on television. I believed I was in a secure location. I felt fully at ease and there was no clear trigger. I suddenly started to experience the signs of a panic attack. My living room's four walls were surrounding me and enclosing me. I felt like I was going to die because I couldn't breathe.

I went outside into my front porch for some fresh air and started practicing deep breathing. Once the symptoms subsided, I began to question why exactly I had that episode. There was no evident cause, no demanding circumstance, and no sign that a panic attack might be about to occur.

The odd thing about panic is that. Your mind can trick you occasionally. Even when you believe there is little chance you may experience a panic attack, your brain may be sensing otherwise. The worrying part is that. The good news is that there are strategies to prevent panic attacks and manage with them considerably better when they occur.

DEALING WITH PANIC ATTACKS

Knowing that you are not the only one who suffers from panic attacks may give you some comfort. Not even one in a million people are you. Nearly 5% of the population in America is thought to have an anxiety disorder of some kind.

Some people may experience only infrequent panic attacks, such as when required to speak in front of others, while others may experience frequent, recurrent panic attacks that prevent them from leaving their homes. Frequently occurring panic attacks frequently result in what doctors refer to as a "anxiety disorder."

Managing an anxiety disorder can be done in a variety of ways. Others might work for you even though some might not. Knowing some of the most popular coping mechanisms can help you deal with panic attacks as soon as they hit.

Knowing when a panic attack is about to start is the first step. Once you've had enough of them, you begin to pay close attention to the tingling sensation, the feeling of being out of breath, and the sense of being disconnected from the world around you.

Many people I speak with are curious about that disconnect. They find it challenging to comprehend. We panic attack sufferers are all too familiar with it. It's similar to being able to see a solid object from a distance. Even though you are aware of its presence, you have some doubts about its veracity.

It's possible that you'll want to touch that thing just to make sure. You feel cut off from the environment around you. It seems as though you have no control over anything around you and are just a spectator in your own life.

This is a terrible feeling, I assure you.

How do you then begin attempting to stop your panic attacks? Would you believe me if I said that the key to stopping panic and anxiety attacks is to WANT one? Doesn't that sound odd, perhaps even contradictory? But the desire actually aids in driving it away. Does this imply that you ought to be able to start having a panic attack right now? Without a doubt! It means that whatever you are afraid of—in this case, a panic attack—will probably manifest and cause havoc. Your chances of repelling the attack increase when you resist it. When you fight against something out of fear, that fear will stay with you. How do you quit resisting? You confront the anxiety head-on, which prevents it from continuing.

In essence, this means that you cannot experience a panic attack if you intentionally seek one out every day. You cannot have a panic attack right now,

I can assure you of that. You may not be aware of it, but you've always chosen to worry. Whether you say this is beyond my power consciously or unconsciously, it is your decision.

Another approach to understand this is to compare experiencing a panic attack to being perched precariously on a precipice. You feel as though the anxiety is bringing you ever closer to losing control. You have to metaphorically jump to get over your fear. You must plunge off the cliff and into all of your greatest fears, including anxiety and fear.

Jumping technique Jumping makes you desire to experience a panic episode. You actively invite anxiety and panic episodes by going about your daily activities.

Your true sense of security comes from knowing that a panic attack can never hurt you. A medical fact is that. Although the feelings are intense, you are protected and nothing bad will happen to you. Although your heart is beating, nothing bad will happen to you. The jump reduces to a two-foot drop only! It's completely secure.

Your life becomes unbalanced as a result of anxiety because of how much mental concern you experience as a top-heavy feeling. Your entire body's center of attention is shifted to your head. Schools of meditation frequently use the ease with which the body can lose its feeling of center as an illustration of this top-heavy imbalance.

Relaxation is the key to conquering panic attacks. It's simple to say but challenging to do that.

Focusing on your breathing and making sure it is slow and steady is a good way to achieve this. Breathing problems are one of the first indications of a panic attack, and you might find yourself panting to take a breath. Your heart rate will slow and the panic will pass if you concentrate on even breathing.

A calming effect of slower, deeper breathing is felt. Letting all of the air out of your lungs will help you breathe more easily. This makes it difficult for your lungs to take a deep breath later. You'll notice that your breathing is deeper and that you feel calmer if you keep your attention on your out-breath and let all the air out of your lungs.

The goal is to divert attention from the fact that you are experiencing a panic attack. One at a time, make an effort to drive your feet into the ground. Feel how firmly anchored to the earth they are.

Lying down with your bottom close to a wall is an even better position. Knees bent, place your feet against the wall, and press each foot into the surface one at a time. It will work better if you can breathe in as you press your foot up against the wall and out as you let go. You ought to switch between your feet. To stop the panic, continue doing this for 10 to 15 minutes.

Consider what you see, hear, feel, and smell in your surroundings by using all of your senses. You'll be able to stay present if you do this. Typically, feelings of panic are connected to unpleasant memories of the past or unpleasant anticipations of the future.

Anything that keeps your attention on the here and now will be soothing. Try holding a pet, scanning your room for colors, textures, and shapes, paying close attention to the sounds you hear, making a friend call, or simply taking in the smells around you.

Aromatherapy is strongly endorsed by many people as a treatment for panic and anxiety. When you smell lavender, it can be especially calming and soothing. Lavender essential oil is widely available in retail outlets. Keep it nearby and inhale when you begin to feel anxious.

Try rubbing some oil (olive or grape seed oil will work) with a few drops of lavender essential oil in it. When not in use, keep a prepared mixture in a dark glass bottle. Even better, prepare multiple bottles, one of which can be small enough to carry around.

Helichrysum, frankincense, and marjoram are further essential oils that have been shown to relieve anxiety and panic episodes. Use the oil that most appeals to you after giving each one a sniff, or a combination of your favorite oils blended with olive or grape seed oil.

You might want to get ready before having a panic attack. Make a list of the things you're worried will happen when you're not in a panic. Then jot down some calming statements that tell you to be afraid of nothing. When terror begins to set in, you might then tell yourself these things.

When you need it, you can refer to your prepared list of things to do in the event of panic. Fill it with numerous calming sayings and suggestions for calming activities. I find this to be a very useful tool, and I never leave home without my little notebook with these encouraging statements in it.

Being in a state of panic can be extremely frightening, especially if you're alone. Making plans for when the panic hits can significantly lessen and occasionally even prevent the panic.

Utilizing visualization is a fantastic additional strategy for reducing stress and anxiety.

USE VISUALIZATION TO RELAX

By using visualization, you can easily release mental tension, stress, and anxious thoughts. When you're under pressure, you can use the visualization, and it's especially helpful when your mind is racing with fearful, anxious thoughts.

When used frequently, this visualization technique is very effective at getting rid of persistent mental anxieties or bothersome thoughts. The exercise must be performed for longer than 10 minutes at a time to reap its full benefits; anything less will not produce discernible effects.

The visualization can be done in any way—there is no right or wrong way. If you feel you are not very good at seeing mental imagery, use your intuition and don't think you can't execute it. You will benefit as long as your focus is on the exercise.

The best place to perform this exercise is in a place where you won't be disturbed. As you gain more experience, you'll be able to achieve the same beneficial effects in a busier setting, like the workplace. Your mental state should become calmer, and you should experience a sense of mental release and relaxation.

Close your eyes and focus on your breath while sitting or standing. Put one hand on your upper chest and the other on your stomach to help you become aware of your breathing. When you breathe in, allow your stomach to expand forward; when you exhale, allow it to gently contract back. Get into a rhythm by breathing consistently at the same depth.

There should be little to no movement in your hand on your chest. Once more, make an effort to inhale at the same depth each time. Diaphragmatic breathing is what is meant by this.

When you're confident with this technique, try to slow down your breathing by taking a brief pause after each exhalation before you take another breath. Although at first it could seem as though you are not breathing deeply enough, continuous practice will eventually make this slower rate feel natural.

Creating a cycle where you count to three when you take a breath in, stop, and then count to three when you exhale (or 2, or 4—whatever is comfortable for you) is frequently beneficial. This will also enable you to concentrate just on breathing without allowing any other thoughts to enter your head.

Simply dismiss any further thoughts that come to mind and return your focus on breathing and counting. For a few minutes, keep doing this. (If you do this often, the diaphragmatic muscle will start to get stronger and function appropriately, giving you a pleasant sense of relaxation all the time.)

Now turn your focus to your feet. Feel your feet as deeply as you can. Test your ability to feel each toe. Imagine roots slowly spreading out through the soles of your feet and descending into the ground. The roots are expanding quickly and penetrating the earth's surface deeply. You feel as secure as a giant oak or redwood tree right now because you are firmly rooted to the ground.

Spend some time focusing on this sense of safety and security that is rooted in the earth. Once you have firmly established the perception or feeling that you are rooted like a tree, see a cloud of brilliant light forming far above you. Your head is struck by a lightning strike from the luminous cloud, which ignites a band of bright white light that slowly descends from your head down your body, over your legs, and out past your toes.

Feel the band of light clearing your mind as it passes over you. Your mind is being illuminated, and any unsettling or stressful thoughts you may have been having are being cleared. Up until you feel a sense of clearing and release from any anxious thinking, repeat this image four or five times.

Finish by picturing yourself standing next to a sizable, glowing waterfall. The water is glistening and teeming with life. You can feel the water running over every part of your body as you stand beneath the waterfall, soothing you and evoking a profound sense of calm within you.

Test the water's flavor. Allow it to cool you off by opening your mouth and allowing it to enter. As it reverberates off the ground all around you, hear it. Your body and mind are being washed clean of tension and worry by the water, which is life itself. You should then open your eyes.

When performing the visualization, make an effort to utilize all of your senses. Use your senses of touch, taste, and hearing to make the images in your head as real as possible. Feel the water trickle down your body and listen to the splashing noise it makes.

You will benefit more if your imagined situations are more realistic. Many people claim that using these straightforward visualizations frequently has very positive and calming effects. The mind is similar to a muscle in that it must periodically let go of what it is holding onto in order to relax.

You can use any setting or circumstance to help you relax. This is compared to "finding your happy place." Perhaps being at the beach or in a pool makes you feel relaxed. Consider going there. Just be sure that wherever you go in your mind, you can find peace and rest.

You are allowing your mind to relax by picturing the various scenarios. Your brain will receive a signal when you close your eyes and start this process that it is time to let go of anything it has been holding onto mentally, including anxious thoughts.

It is crucial to do this every day in order to train

your mind to release stress. You can learn to release all stress minutes after beginning the exercise with practice. You should do your daily practice right before bed because it will help you sleep better at night.

Many people perform these visualizations before going to bed in a different room than their bedroom. In this manner, individuals leave the mental stress and worrisome thoughts behind them when they enter the bedroom and shut the door. Just make sure you have the chance to fully focus on your inner visions.

It is quite useful to use visualization as a stress management technique. If this vision is done correctly, you can experience a profound sense of inner tranquility. This method can help prevent an anxiety attack from starting, but it is unlikely to be effective in stopping one. It is a really effective strategy for helping you get rid of feelings of general worry.

With practice, you discover that you may go days without having worried thoughts interfere with your life. This is crucial because it dramatically lowers the amount of overall anxiety you experience.

Simply said, visualization is a skill you can employ to combat anxious thoughts and feelings. Let's examine several strategies for reducing excessive stress, starting with music.

BEAT STRESS WITH MUSIC

Music can do wonders for reducing stress. Everyone has different musical preferences. The music that makes us feel at ease should be played. Stress may not be reduced by forcing yourself to sit down and listen to music for relaxation that you dislike. The impact of music as a mood enhancer and stress reliever is significant and multifaceted.

Sounds have a significant impact on the entire energetic system of the human body; certain tones and frequencies have a particular effect on the physical body and chakra centers. The benefits of someone actually playing or creating music themselves should receive extra attention.

Increased deep breathing is one of the first stress-reduction changes that happen when we hear music. Serotonin synthesis in the body also quickens.

It has been discovered that playing background music while we work, seemingly unaware of the music itself, helps to lessen workplace stress. To distract you from the high prices, many retail locations play music while you shop.

Music was found to lower heart rates and increase body temperature, which is a sign that relaxation is beginning. Relaxation therapy alone was less effective than relaxation therapy combined with music.

Many experts contend that, despite our lack of awareness of it, the rhythm or beat of the music is what has the calming effect on us. They make the observation that we were probably influenced by our mother's heartbeat when we were infants in the womb. Later in life, we react to the calming music, probably because it reminds us of our mother's nurturing, relaxing surroundings.

One of the most calming or nerve-wracking experiences is listening to music. It can be challenging to decide what will work for an individual; most people choose to go with what they "enjoy" rather than what might be helpful.

Many unexpected things were discovered after conducting considerable research on the effects that any particular piece of music has on the physiological response system. In reality, several of the so-called meditation and relaxation recordings led to unfavorable EEG patterns that were on par with those of heavy metal and hard rock.

The surprising part was how calming a lot of Celtic, Native American, and other music genres with loud drums or flutes were. The most important discovery was that any music played live, even at moderate volume levels and even if it was a little discordant, had a very positive effect.

As we previously stated, not one type of music is suitable for everyone. Individuals have varying tastes. It's crucial that you enjoy the tunes being played. A recent rest and relaxation CD I purchased from Wal-Mart has worked wonders for me. It plays lovely piano music with the sound of the ocean in the background. It is very calming.

One thing to keep in mind: If you're trying to unwind, it's probably not a good idea to listen to certain ballads or songs that conjure up sad memories for you. The cause is clear. You're making an effort to unwind and get rid of your worrying thoughts. The last thing you want is for a depressing tune to trigger unwanted memories.

Here are some broad recommendations for using music to reduce stress.

• Try taking a 20-minute "sound bath" to relieve tension. Play some soothing music on your stereo, then find a comfortable spot on a couch or the floor close to the speakers and lie down. You can wear headphones for a more immersive experience to help you concentrate and cut out outside distractions.

• Listen to music with a rhythm that is slower than your heart's normal rate of 72 beats per minute. Most people have found that repetitive or cyclical music is effective.

•

Allow the music to wash over you as it plays, washing away your day's stress. Concentrate on your breathing and allow it to slow down, deepen, and become regular. Focus on the space between the notes in the music to avoid overanalyzing it and to further your state of relaxation.

•

After a long day at work, faster music will be more stimulating than slow, relaxing music. AVOID SILENCE and DANCE! Whether or if you can dance well is unimportant. Simply follow the music and do what feels right. The sense of release will astound you!

•

When times are bad, turn to familiar music, such as an old favorite or a childhood favorite. Often, familiarity fosters serenity.

• Use the walkman to go for walks while listening to your favorite music. Breathe in and out in time with the music. Give up to the music's pull. With the help of music, images, and movement (a brisk walk), this is a fantastic way to reduce stress.

• You can lessen tension by listening to natural noises like ocean waves or the stillness of a dense forest. If you're close to a peaceful area of forests or the sea, consider going for a 15 to 20 minute walk. If not, numerous music stores sell recordings of these sounds. I've found this to be quite peaceful, and you should too!

Self-hypnosis is a fantastic relaxation technique that I have discovered to help me deal with my personal anxiety issues.

FREE OF STRESS WITH SELF-HYPNOSIS

I remember feeling particularly stressed and anxious a few weeks ago. Everything that could go wrong, it seemed, did. I had the impression that I was losing control. I stumbled upon a website offering a downloadable mp3 hypnotic relaxation session while I was writing a book on yoga and meditation at the time. It was the best $20 I've ever spent, and it only cost me about $20! These downloadable sessions are available for a small fee in many locations on the internet. Self-hypnosis is a technique that you can learn on your own as well. Finding a calm environment where you can unwind completely and hear your inner voice is the first step. Never try to force something to happen. Relax and listen with your mind free. Allowing that hypnotic state to develop naturally is key to achieving it. Additionally, avoid looking out for any indications that you might be hypnotized. We can assure you that if you watch out for these warning signs, you won't be able to fully unwind and enjoy the self-hypnosis benefits.

Hypnosis can be experienced in a variety of ways. Nobody's experience will be the same for everyone. But there is one thing that everyone agrees on: being hypnotized is always enjoyable! In hypnosis, there are no "bad trips." Keep in mind that self-hypnosis is a skill that you can develop, and as you do, it gets stronger and stronger.

Setting up a practice routine is an excellent idea. Depending on how busy you are and how much time you have available, allow yourself anywhere from 10 to 30 minutes. If you can, practice when your day is most enjoyable and when you are least likely to be bothered by other people.

The majority of people find it most effective to practice lying down in a relaxed setting with the fewest distractions possible. You might try to hide the noise with another source of sound if it bothers you while you are practicing.

If you like, play stereo music or white noise in the background. Try switching the stations on your radio receiver if, like the majority of people, you don't have a white noise maker. When you do that, you get static that sounds like white noise. However, this requires a non-noise-canceling FM receiver that is older or less expensive. AM tuners can be used for this occasionally. This shouldn't be too loud to be distracting; it should just be in the background.

Relaxation, deepening, application of suggestions, and termination make up the four main parts of a hypnotic induction.1. Relaxation

Your first job in the hypnotic induction is to slow the juices down and get yourself relaxed. But don't try to force your mind to relax (whatever that means)! If you get yourself physically relaxed, your mind will follow.

Relaxation – really deep relaxation – is an ability that most people have either lost or never developed. Some people can do it quite easily, though. They just let go of their tensions and let every part of their body become limp and relaxed. If you are one of these people, begin your self-hypnosis practice by getting nicely relaxed. Take your time. This is not something you want to rush.

The time involved for the relaxation phase of your self-hypnosis induction can vary from half an hour to just a few seconds. It is an important part of the induction and should not be slighted. As you get better and your skill increases you will recognize deeply relaxed states, and you will be able to achieve them in a surprisingly short time. But as a beginner, take your time. It will be time well spent.

A very popular method of deep relaxation is the Jacobson Progressive Relaxation procedure. This involves tensing each of the major muscle groups of your body (foot and lower leg on each side, upper leg and hip, abdomen, etc.). Tense the muscle group for a few seconds, then let go.

2. Deepening Procedures

You can start to deepen the relaxed state once you have finished the relaxation phase of your self-hypnosis induction procedure. You will enter a hypnotic state at some point between the deep relaxation and the deepening procedures. It will happen eventually, even if you are a beginner, you just won't know it.

One of the first challenges a newcomer faces is the urge to "watch for it." That is, you will continue to wait for hypnosis to occur, for some alteration in your awareness or your sensations to indicate to you that you are under hypnosis.

If you don't get the thought of watching for hypnosis out of your head, it will undoubtedly get in the way. In this way, entering a hypnotic trance is similar to falling asleep. You are much less likely to fall asleep if you try to catch yourself doing it—if you try to be aware of the precise second that you do fall asleep. You can't sleep while "watching."

In a similar manner, you won't be able to recognize when you enter a hypnotic state (although you won't be able to because you won't have lost consciousness). Later, after a few weeks or months of consistent practice, you'll be much more familiar with yourself and how being hypnotized feels.

Does everyone require weeks or even months to reach a good trance state? Absolutely not. Some people experience it for the first time in an amazing way. Others may practice for a few days without noticing anything, and then all of a sudden have one of those great induction sessions during which they suddenly realize something extraordinarily positive occurred. However, if you're not one of them, don't stress about it. You'll succeed if you just keep working at it.

The count-down approach is one of the most widely used deepening techniques. This one is also popular in Hollywood. That explains why it appears in so many films. Along with the watch that swings.

Simply begin counting down from, say, 20, to employ the count-down approach (or 100, or whatever). After some practice, change the countdown number to whatever seems comfortable to you. Imagine that with each count, you are descending more. As you count, more images and ideas will likely enter your head. That makes sense. Continue counting while you kindly sweep them aside.

You should count down at a natural pace that is neither too fast nor too sluggish. For the majority of people, this entails counting roughly every two or three seconds. Work at a pace that is easy and comfortable for you. Some individuals like to relate the count to breathing. Their breathing slows down as they float deeper, which causes their counting to slow down as well.

Just mentally work your way down the count; don't count aloud. You want to limit your physical activity and movement as much as possible.

3. Suggestion Application in self-hypnosis

Once you have reached the end of your deepening procedure you are ready to apply suggestions. What you have done during the relaxation and deepening procedures is increase your suggestibility. That is, you have opened up your subconscious mind at least a little bit to receive your suggestions. This works because of the particular, and peculiar, characteristics of the subconscious part of your mind.

The most common and easiest way to apply suggestions is to have them worked out ahead of time, properly prepared and worded, and memorized. It should not be too difficult to remember them because they should be rather short and you are the one who composed them. If you have them ready and remembered, you can simply think your way through them at this point.

Dialogue, or more properly monologue, is also okay. You just talk ("think" to keep your effort to a minimum) to yourself about what it is you want to do, be, become, whatever.

Don't say "you." You are thinking to yourself, so use the first person personal pronoun "I." Some suggestions can be succinctly stated in a somewhat more formal sort of way, like, "I am eating less and becoming more slender every day."

Elaborated suggestions are generally wordier and more of an ad lib: "Food is becoming less important to me every day and I am filling my time with more important and meaningful pursuits than eating. It is getting easier and easier to pass up desserts and other fattening foods . . ." and so on.

Generally speaking, the most effective kind of suggestion is image suggestion. Image suggestions usually do not use language at all. You can liken this to seeing yourself in a calm, relaxed state while in the middle of a chaotic situation. Actually see yourself in your mind's eye.

Although people sometimes see immediate results from their suggestions, it is more likely to take a little time for them to kick in. So don't be impatient. On the other hand, if you have not begun to see some results within, say, a couple of weeks, you need to change your suggestions.

4. Termination

You have completed your induction when you have finished implementing the suggestions, at which point you can end the session. You could simply open your eyes, stand up, and carry on with your day, but that is not recommended.

The conclusion of every session should be declared in writing. By doing this, you establish a distinct separation between your normal conscious awareness and the hypnotic state. Additionally, a clear end to your self-hypnosis practice session stops it from morphing into a nap. Take a nap if you feel like it. However, avoid doing it in a way that links practicing self-hypnosis with sleeping.

It's acceptable to practice before going to sleep if you don't care if you stay asleep. Draw the boundary for the end of your self-hypnosis session nonetheless.

Think to yourself that you will be fully awake and alert after you count up to, say, three to end the session.

"One, I'm starting to emerge from it and am heading

toward waking up. Two, I'm starting to wake up and am becoming more awake. Third, I'm fully awake." equivalent to that

When self-hypnosis is used frequently, it can be very effective. You'd be astonished at the degree of relaxation you can get. One of the best things I've ever done for myself, I should add.

We should now discuss general stress management strategies. This chapter may be lengthy, but it is quite beneficial.

STRESS MANAGEMENT

1.Stress is a part of life,

as we have previously stated. Nothing can be done to avoid it. Actually, some stress is beneficial. You might not believe it, but occasionally stress can inspire us to take actions that we might not typically take when we're calm. When we are under stress, we can muster the courage to act when we ordinarily might hesitate. In order to successfully manage stress and allow it to improve our lives rather than control them, we need to be resilient. How can one become tough and resilient? By learning how to manage your stress and turn it into an asset rather than a liability.

Recognizing stress symptoms can be helpful because it motivates us to act, and the sooner the better. The death of a loved one, the birth of a child, a job promotion, or the beginning of a new relationship are some of the more frequent events that cause those emotions. However, it's not always simple to determine why you feel stressed in each situation. As we restructure our lives, we feel stress.

When you experience these signs of stress, your body is pleading with you to assist it. In this chapter, we're going to make a lot of recommendations for you. We're willing to bet that some of them will, even though not all of them will work for you. To manage stress, there are three main strategies. The first is an approach that focuses on action. With this approach, the issues that lead to stress are identified, and the appropriate adjustments are made for a life free of stress.

The following strategy is emotionally focused, and in it, the person manages stress by providing the situation that stressed them a new perspective. The stressful circumstance is viewed in a humorous or alternative light.

I particularly support this method of stress reduction. If you don't laugh at a scenario, you might start sobbing hysterically sometimes. That is not a remedy. So train your eyes to perceive laughter rather than gloom.

The third strategy is an acceptance-focused strategy. This strategy focuses on handling tension that was brought on by a former issue.

The first stress-reduction advice is to identify the underlying causes of your stress. Nobody knows your issue better than you do. Spending a few minutes to identify your true emotions can completely alter the situation.

Determine the cause of the stress during this process. Share it with a loved one nearby if they are present. Take a deep breath and count to ten if you are feeling overly overwhelmed and on the verge of collapsing. This revitalizes the entire body by pumping more oxygen into it.

When under extreme stress, take a moment to meditate and step outside of the immediate environment. From your current position, get up and start walking. Attempt to stretch. You'll soon notice that the stress has subsided.

This is due to the fact that you are currently calm, which is the best stress reliever. Another technique for managing stress is to smile. Simply get up and grin at your coworker in the opposite corner if you're at work. Your mood will alter, you'll notice. Pick up some basic yoga or meditation skills.

You can also come up with your own stress-reduction strategies. The fundamental concept is to pinpoint the source of stress, take a break from it for a while, and then address it. Another method of reducing stress is to take a quick stroll while admiring natural objects. Simple stress-reduction techniques include drinking a glass of water and playing quick games. The aim is to shift your attention away from the issue so that when you return to it, it won't seem as overwhelming as it did before. You may reduce stress by following these five short steps: 1. Don't just sit there. Move! Many psychologists believe that motion elicits emotion. You could have noticed that it's simpler to get depressed when you're not doing anything. You droop in a chair, lowering your heart rate, decreasing the amount of oxygen getting to your brain, and preventing air from getting to your lungs. Regardless of how you are feeling right now, I dare you to get up and move quickly. Perhaps you should enter a room that is unoccupied and hop around a little bit. Although it may seem absurd, the outcomes speak for themselves. Right away, give it a try. It works enchantment.

A fantastic way to reduce stress is to exercise. A panic episode during aerobic activity may scare those with anxiety disorders. After all, as you exercise, your breathing gets heavier, your heart rate increases, and you start sweating.

It's not an attack, so don't freak out! While you are working out, keep telling yourself this. Recognize that there is a significant distinction between what happens when you workout and the physical side of it.

2. Take in the roses.

How do you take a whiff of roses? Consider making an investment to fund the vacation you've always wanted to take. Visit an exotic location-rich nation to spark your imagination and inspire your creativity. You must step away from your routine and travel a little.

3. Assist others in solving their challenges.

When you immerse yourself in helping others, it is immensely soothing. You'd be shocked at how many people have issues that are more serious than yours. There are various ways in which you can help others. Don't let stress and depression cause you to cuddle up in bed.

Get outside and assist someone. But take care. Avoid getting sucked into other people's issues in an effort to ignore your own.

Friends and family call me frequently when they need to vent or seek advise. Don't call the "crazy" person for advice, I jokingly advise. However, there are times when I find myself worrying about the people who call me and I become preoccupied with their problems. I find that I need to take a break and reevaluate my priorities because this only adds to my already high level of stress.

Now I can tell them to call back later because I'm just not able to handle it right now. They occasionally become upset, but more often than not, they comprehend. I've learned, though, not to let their responses get to me. It should matter now even if it won't matter in a week.

4. Have a little fun.

You've probably already heard that laughter is a healthy internal remedy. It relaxes the muscles and releases tension. Blood starts to flow to the heart and brain as a result. More importantly, laughing causes the release of a substance that relieves pain in the body.

Researchers learn new advantages of laughter every day. Can you occasionally benefit from a good dose of belly-shaking laughter? You can, of course. What are you holding out for? Rent some amusing movies or visit a comedy club.

5. Exhaust your knees.

If I could give you one lasting solution when things get rough, it would be prayer. Depending on their religion, many individuals may refer to it as meditation. What you call it doesn't matter to me as long as you have somewhere to flee to.

You now have a few options for immediate stress relief. Need more? No issue!

BONUS TIPS (STRESS MANAGEMENT)

1.Make anxiety your friend.

Make stress your buddy and acknowledge its benefits! The body's natural "fight or flight" response will cause that energy burst to improve your performance when it matters most. A top athlete who was completely at ease before a major competition has yet to be seen. When it matters most, use stress to your advantage and push yourself a little bit harder.

2. Stress spreads easily

This means that negative people can cause a lot of stress. Stress is bred by negativity, and some people only know how to complain. Now, there are two ways to approach this. They hope that you can help them get back "up" because they first perceive you as a positive, upbeat person. If not, they are simply a pessimistic individual who is unable to feel better about themselves unless those around them share their viewpoints.

Avoid getting sucked into their behavior of downing. Limit your contact with these people after realizing that they deal with stress on their own. You could try to play stress doctor and teach them better stress management techniques, but tread carefully as this could increase your own stress levels more.

3. Model stress-management skills

Who remains composed when everyone else is losing their cool? What exactly are they changing? What attitude do they have? What dialect do they speak? Are they skilled and knowledgeable?

Determine it from a distance or have a conversation with them. Study the most effective stress-reducers and do as they say.

4. Take deep breaths.

By breathing deeply, you can deceive your body into relaxing. Take a slow seven-count inhalation and an eleven-count exhalation. Repeat the 7-11 breathing exercise until your heart rate decreases, your sweat-covered hands stop, and you begin to feel more normal.

5. Stop worrying thoughts

You could get yourself all by yourself into a stress knot. "If this occurs, that may occur, and then we're all in deep water!" Why waste all that energy worrying needlessly when the majority of these things never happen?

Give stressful thoughts the red light and put a stop to them. Okay, so there's a chance that something could go wrong. How likely is that, and what can you do to avoid it?

6. Recognize your stress triggers and hot areas

delivering challenging comments, dealing with clients, presenting presentations, meeting deadlines, etc. The mere act of penning them down has my heart racing.

Make a list of your own stress hot spots or trigger points. Be precise. Do presentations to particular audiences tend to rile you up more than others? Do certain projects stress people out more than others? Have you consumed too much coffee?

Knowing what makes you stressed out is useful information because you can take steps to reduce your stress. Do you need to pick up any new abilities? Are additional resources required? Should you switch to decaffeinated coffee instead?

7. Fill up on food, drink, rest, and joy!

Our body and mind suffer greatly when we are sleep deprived, eat poorly, or do not exercise. Kind of obvious, but important to highlight because it's frequently overlooked as a stress-reduction method. Don't burn the candle at both ends; instead, pay attention to your mother!

Stay away from artificial stress relief methods. This means that you shouldn't instinctively pour a drink of wine or smoke a cigarette when you feel yourself starting to become agitated. Actually, substances like alcohol, cigarettes, caffeine, and narcotics can exacerbate the issue. Practice the relaxing methods we've given you instead would be a better option.

You can then have that glass of wine if you'd like once you're at ease.

8. Take in the beauty of nature outside.

A little sunshine and exercise can have a remarkable impact on your stress level and improve your outlook on life as a whole. Everyone in your family and/or circle of friends will benefit from your improved attitude, and problems that initially seemed overwhelming will fade into insignificance, leaving you wondering what the problem was.

You won't just feel less stressed; you'll also be better for it—healthier, happier, and more energized—and prepared to take on any challenges that come your way.

9. Permit yourself to revert to your childlike state.

What did you like to do as a kid? Be imaginative; draw, paint, etc. Play around dance, play-dough, or reading. Play some music and express yourself without worrying about conforming to society's expectations of who you "should" be. Just unwind and have fun. We all have a little child inside of us, and it's a good idea to occasionally let that child out to play.

If I may say so, this suggestion is great and extremely healing. I can speak from experience. Nothing makes me happier than purchasing a brand-new box of 64 Crayons—the kind with the sharpener inside the box—and coloring endlessly in a coloring book. When I use this stress reliever, my grandson loves it!

10. Avoid setting yourself up for failure by doing so.

By giving ourselves unattainable goals, many of us unwittingly set ourselves up for failure. Realize that you cannot lose 40 pounds in just one or two months, for instance, if you are dieting.

Or perhaps your goal is to obtain a specific job position; whatever your objective, give yourself enough time to accomplish it and be aware that setbacks occasionally happen.

You will feel even better about yourself if you accomplish your objective without encountering any obstacles, but don't count on it. In actuality, don't have any expectations; reality frequently differs greatly from expectations.

11. Recognize that occasionally saying "no" is acceptable.

Many of us frequently feel that we must always respond positively to requests for assistance and feel that we must always say "yes" to everyone. But keep in mind that you cannot please everyone. Before you can fully offer others what they need while keeping yourself happy, you must first take care of your own needs.

12. You are not required to comply with all requests from your family, friends, and others.

Yes, you should assist others, but only after you have taken the necessary steps to look after yourself.

13. Give yourself the priority
that it deserves;

once your needs are addressed, you'll find that you have more time for others. And if you don't feel that you have to continually put other people's needs ahead of your own, you might enjoy helping others more. We're still not done! There are countless effective methods for overcoming stress and anxiety. You have a right to learn everything you can. After all, isn't it the main reason you're reading this book? Here are some other stress relievers.

WHO YU GUNNA CALL?
STRESS BUSTERS!

1.I've personally used this idea a
lot and really love it!

Yell! Yes, scream as loudly as you can, at the top of your lungs. Even though you might not be able to do this at home, it works perfectly when you're driving with the windows down. yelled guttural from the bottom of my soul. It liberates you!

2. Sing.

As we mentioned in the previous chapter, listening to music can be a very effective way to relieve stress. Imagine how much better you'll feel if you sing "Copacabana" loud and proud! Who gives a damn if you can't sing? You're pursuing this for yourself!

3. Start a new activity,

such as knitting or crocheting. Don't stress about doing it well. The process itself is advantageous. For many people, remaining motionless while performing repetitive movements is calming and stabilizing. It might be time for you to gather your thoughts.

Start a garden,

4. Apartment residents can also accomplish this

. Potted plants can be found inside, outside, or in a small area of your yard. It takes a little effort to set up.

It's rewarding to take care of plants, fruits, veggies, and flowers and watch them grow, bloom, or provide food. The best approach to manage tension and concern, according to ardent gardeners, is to work in the garden. The improvement of the environment's beauty and tranquility is a bonus.

5. Have fun with a cat or dog. According to experts, pet owners live longer and have fewer signs of stress than non-pet owners. Playing with your pet is healthy for both you and the animal! It's a sort of social connection where you're not under any obligation to please anyone!

6. Take a look at the moon and stars. Observing the night sky while lying on a blanket with your hands behind your head may be incredibly humbling. It's not just humble; it's also incredibly lovely and soothing.

My grandson and I recently spread a blanket out in the yard to watch the moon set behind the clouds and to look at the stars. Seeing the sky through his eyes made it even more intriguing for me. He is only three years old, so it is a great experience for him.

We talked about astronauts who get to view the stars up close and how the universe is vast while we are still so small, and I felt all my anxieties wash away. The vastness of the sky makes you realize how insignificant our troubles are in comparison. Seeing that one bright star in the sky that is always above my house gives me a lot of comfort as well.

After leaving the funeral for my best friend's mother, we got out of the car and I paused to look at the stars with my friend's five-year-old. "That's my grandma," she replied, pointing to a certain star. She is now our protector angel. I can always count on Cheryl to get me through anything when I see that star.

JUST SAY NO!

The ability to say "No" when necessary is a huge issue for people who are overly stressed. Perhaps your mother wants you to take Grandma to the store, but you're working on a significant project at work right now. When you've already made plans with yourself to get a haircut, perhaps your best friend asks if you'd mind watching her children. You are not required to accept everyone's invitations. In fact, there are numerous occasions when you should decline their invitations. You are a people pleaser if you frequently find yourself saying "yes" to requests that you really don't want to make. Although this isn't a bad trait in general, it can be extremely stressful.

People-pleasers put the needs of others ahead of their own. They spend a lot of time serving the needs of others and worry constantly about what they want, think, or need. They rarely take care of their own needs and feel bad when they do. Being a people-pleaser is challenging.

People-pleasers are reluctant to express their true opinions or request what they need because they fear offending others. However, they frequently interact with people who are completely uninterested in their needs. In fact, people-pleasers frequently feel compelled to cheer up insensitive or unhappy people, even at their own expense.

It is exhausting to constantly try to please others, and many people pleasers frequently experience feelings of anxiety, worry, unhappiness, and fatigue. Even though they give so much to others and may not understand why they receive nothing in return, they frequently refuse to ask for what they require.

This is the trap I got caught in. Every time I offered to help someone else, I discovered that when I needed those same folks to assist ME, they were mysteriously preoccupied.

A people-pleaser might think that if they ask for assistance and the other person agrees, they are only doing it out of obligation and not out of genuine desire. It is believed that if they truly intended to assist, they would have done it without my request.

This style of thinking develops because people-pleasers themselves feel obligated to lend a hand and don't always act out of pure motivation. Unfortunately, people-pleasers have been taught that their value is based on what they do for other people.

Being a people pleaser is painful—trust me, I know! People-pleasers frequently take things personally, are very sensitive to other people's feelings, and rarely put their own needs first.

They are frequently on the go, rushing to complete tasks because when they do take some time for themselves, they feel egotistical, indulgent, and guilty. People pleasers are often the first to be asked to do things, which makes them vulnerable to being exploited because they accomplish so much and are easy to get along with.

Most likely, people pleasers were raised in households where their needs and feelings were not valued, respected, or given much weight. When they were young, they frequently had to meet or tend to the needs of others. Alternatively, they might have been silenced, neglected, or subjected to other forms of abuse, learning that their needs and feelings were unimportant.

Girls are taught in many cultures to be people-pleasers who put the needs of others before their own. There is at least some element of people-pleasing in many women. Men who related to their mothers frequently did so as well.

People pleasers tend to put more of their attention on others than on themselves. They frequently feel empty or are unsure of their feelings, thoughts, or personal goals. However, it is possible to break this pattern and improve your self-esteem. I was able to figure out how to stop this cycle. If you identify with the above description, you can take the same action. You're curious about how. It's simpler than you might imagine! Practice saying no first. This word is very significant! Just to hear the word come out of your mouth, repeat it as often as you can. When you are by yourself, say it aloud. Practice saying "No, I can't do that" or "No, I don't want to go there," among other NO-containing sentences. Try it out for easy situations first, and work your way up to more challenging ones.

You shouldn't constantly say "yes." Prior to responding to someone's request, try pausing or taking a deep breath. The phrase "I need to think about it first, I'll get back to you" or "Let me check my schedule and call you back" are possible responses to requests. Use any term that gives you time before automatically answering "YES" and that you feel comfortable using.

Take brief pauses, despite your guilt. Although you won't constantly feel guilty, you probably will at first. Keep in mind that the annoyance you might have to endure from others is well worth maintaining your mental wellness. You are what's crucial. Everyone around you will be healthy if you are!

Find out what makes you happy. For instance, you might enjoy listening to music, visiting parks, viewing videos, or reading periodicals. Give yourself the go-ahead to do such things, then take pleasure in them.

Request assistance from someone. Although I realize it's challenging, you can accomplish it! Why shouldn't YOU ask THEM if everyone else is asking YOU for favors? Just be understanding if they reject you. Simply because you've always said "yes," doesn't mean they have to reciprocate.

Become aware of your thoughts and feelings. These things are significant to be aware of since they define who you are. Then, try expressing your thoughts and feelings more frequently. Just be mindful to maintain some civility when necessary.

Many people-pleasers think that if they stop doing things for other people, no one would like them. You're being used by someone if they stop liking you because you refuse to do what they ask, and you probably don't want them as a friend anyway.

People will like you not just for what you do, but also for who you are. You have the right to put yourself first, to refuse requests from others, and to take care of yourself without feeling guilty. One little step at a time, you can make a change.

The majority of people, I believe, would agree wholeheartedly with what I have to say next. McDonald's was right when they said, "You Deserve A Break Today!

TAKE A BREAK

So often, we know inside ourselves that we need a break. That break might be a full-fledged vacation or a weekend getaway. Either way, getting out of the daily grind can be amazingly liberating and a huge way to get rid of stress and anxiety.

Unfortunately, many people think they can't take the time to get away. This is toxic thinking. Get out and get away!

How many times have you continued working, knowing that you are not giving 100% to the task at hand? How many times have you read or written the same sentence over and over again, as your mind keeps wandering and thinking about other things? How often have you wanted to take a break from the family or kids but feared the consequences of doing so? It's time for a break!

Why do we not allow ourselves the time to take a 'time out'? Perhaps we feel like we don't deserve it or that there's just too much to be done. There are many genuine reasons for needing to complete jobs and tasks; however we may also on occasion have 'hidden agendas' as to why we cannot stop for a break. Why?

It could be ego. Some people simply enjoy boasting

about, 'how late they had to work in order to complete a project' or 'how much effort they invested in order to complete the job so quickly'. This type of person is often looking to impress others with their efforts, thereby increasing their ego in the process.

Maybe you think you just can't take the time off. "I can't stop; I just have to get this finished". Does this sound familiar? "I can't stop because the job has to be finished, WHY? So I can move straight on to the next thing, and the next, and the next etc..." This person will find that there is always something that has to be done, which will constantly prevent him/ her from taking a break.

Maybe you just feel like you need to be needed. A mother managing the household, kids and other chores may feel as if her household will collapse if she were to put her feet up or take a weekend off! By not taking a break she can keep convincing herself that her role is crucial and the family would collapse without her input. This may indeed be true, but is still not a good enough reason to prevent her having a rest!

Get rid of that thinking! You can get some amazing benefits just by taking a little time for yourself! Allowing your mind and/or body to rest can help re-focus your attention, sharpen your wits and increase motivation. In addition, taking time out helps to relieve stress, can aid the recovery of tired muscles and also promotes the discovery that there is more to life than just work.

Many athletes will tell you that an important part of their training routine is rest. Muscles need time to repair after a workout. Remember that your brain is a type of muscle as well. It needs time to rest and recuperate in order to perform at its best. By giving your brain time off, you'll be able to better concentrate and give tasks you once found difficult your full attention. They'll be easier, believe me!

So you've decided that a break is in order. Good for you! A break can be anything from a 10-minute meditation session to a trip around the world, and anything in-between. I think a break should be something that takes your mind off of a preoccupation with the everyday tedium of life.

So depending on the time you wish to avail towards relaxing you may enjoy reading, watching a movie, cooking, playing with the kids, riding a motorbike or driving, exercising or doing sports, traveling or simply sleeping!

While you are taking this rest, above all, allow yourself the time to do it and don't feel guilty about. You will gain so very much by this time off, so enjoy the time you are giving yourself.

Life will go on without you and contrary to what your mind might be telling you, everyone will survive – even when you're not there! Let everything go and concentrate on YOU for once instead of everyone around you!

If you're feeling tired, unmotivated or just in need of a rest, don't be a martyr or look negatively at this. You may actually find that in reality, allowing yourself a break will actually help you ultimately become more efficient and effective in every part of your life. Plus you'll get the badly needed recharging of your "batteries" that you need and sorely deserve! Work can probably be one of the most stressful places to be. You might think that none of these techniques can help you when you're around your co-workers. You couldn't be more wrong.

RELAXING
AT WORK

Coffee breaks aren't the only times when you can take a moment for yourself. Experience has actually taught me that coffee (or smoke) breaks can actually add to the stress you feel when you're at work.

Some of the suggestions we've given you in this book can certainly be practiced at work, but, unfortunately, others cannot. Here's a tried and true method to help you relax at work.

First and foremost, find a place to sit. Sit up straight with your back against the back of your chair, your feet flat on the floor, and your hands resting lightly on your thighs.

If possible, close your eyes. You may do the exercise without closing your eyes, but closing your eyes will help you relax a bit more. Do not clench your eyes shut. Let your eyelids fall naturally.

Breathe in slowly through your nose, counting to 5. Hold the breath for a count of 5. Breathe out slowly, counting to five. Repeat.

This exercise is performed by tensing and holding a

set of muscles for a count of 5, and then relaxing the set of muscles for a count of 5.

When you tense each muscle set, do it as hard as you can without hurting yourself. When you release the hold, be as relaxed as possible.

Begin by tensing your feet. Do this by pulling your feet off the floor and your toes toward you while keeping your heels on the floor. Hold for a slow count of 5. Release the hold. Let your feet fall gently back. Feel the relaxation. Think about how it feels compared to when you tensed the muscles. Relax for a count of 5.

Next tense your thigh muscles as hard as you can. Hold for a count of 5. Relax the muscles and count to 5.

Tighten your abdominal muscles and hold for a count of 5. Relax the muscles for a count of 5. Be sure you are continuing to sit up straight.

Tense your arm and hand muscles by squeezing your hands into fists as hard as you can. Hold for a count of 5. Relax the muscles completely for a count of 5.

Tighten your upper back by pushing your shoulders back as if you are trying to touch your shoulder blades together. Hold for a count of 5. Relax for a count of 5.

Tense your shoulders by raising them toward your ears as if shrugging and holding for a count of 5. Relax for a count of 5.

Tighten your neck first by gently moving your head back (as if looking at the ceiling) and holding for 5.

Relax for 5. Then gently drop your head forward and hold for 5. Relax for a count of 5.

Tighten your face muscles. First open your mouth wide and hold for 5. Relax for 5. Then raise your eye brows up high and hold for 5. Relax for 5. Finally clench your eyes tightly shut and hold for 5. Relax (with eyes gently closed) for 5.

Finish the exercise with breathing. Breathe in slowly through your nose, counting to 5. Hold the breath for a count of 5. Breathe out slowly, counting to five. Repeat 4 times. And that's it!

Perform this exercise whenever you need to relax, whether it's on a plane or in a car or anyplace else you may be sitting. Because this exercise may be very relaxing, it should not be performed while driving.

Over time, if performed regularly, this exercise will help you recognize tension in your body. You will be able to relax muscles at any time rather than performing the entire exercise. Perform at least twice a day for long-term results.

You may develop your own longer relaxation exercise by adding more muscle groups. Pinpoint your own areas of tension then tense and relax these areas in the same way.

Maximize the relaxation benefits of this exercise by visualizing a peaceful scene at the end of the exercise. Visualize a scene - a place where you feel relaxed - in detail for at least 5 minutes. Remember the happy place? Go there and enjoy it!

CONCLUSION

We hope you realize and comprehend that there is NO WAY to completely eliminate stress from your life if you take nothing else away from reading this book. What you can do is figure out how to use that stress to your advantage. It's not as difficult to manage stress as it may appear. But we cannot stress this next point enough. Consult your physician, a spiritual guide, or a local mental health organization if you feel that your life is too stressful. They might advise you to consult a psychiatrist, psychologist, social worker, or other qualified counselor because responses to stress can play a role in depression, anxiety, and other disorders. We don't want to come across as experts in medicine. All we're trying to do is give you some tools you can use to deal with the things that overwhelm and make us feel out of control in your life. To reduce some of your stress, you might also want to look into time management tools. You definitely don't want to experience anxiety if you feel like you don't have enough time to complete the tasks at hand. This increases stress. Simple, inexpensive strategies to effectively reduce stress include stress management techniques. They can be used at any time and anywhere. Well, nearly! Do not hesitate to seek assistance if you think you need it. You might not always be right. Your stress may be coming from absolutely nothing. But its origins could be physical. It might be a simple problem for someone else to resolve. Recognizing your limitations can significantly reduce stress.

The stress of everyday life is common. Stress is beneficial in moderation because it can spur motivation and increase output. But excessive stress or a strong reaction to stress can be harmful.

It can make you more susceptible to both general ill health and particular physical or mental conditions like infection, heart disease, or depression. Stress that is constant and unrelenting can cause anxiety as well as unhealthy habits like overeating and drug or alcohol abuse.

The things that relieve stress vary from person to person, just as the causes of stress do. However, most people find it helpful to make some lifestyle adjustments and to find pleasurable, healthy ways to deal with stress. I hope I've given you some excellent strategies for coping with the stress we all experience!

Above all, keep in mind that you are not fighting this battle by yourself. There are countless numbers of people who feel absolutely out of control and overwhelmed. We wanted to send you this book for that reason. So that you might discover inner peace and understand why everyone is on this great blue marble.

Also, you are! Live life to the fullest and take it all in. And when you experience stress or a panic attack, remember to breathe through it and to relax since a great many other people can relate to how you're feeling.

"Don't Worry, Be Happy.